Aromatherapy: The Healthy Complete Guide to Essential Oils

What You Need To Know About Aromatherapy

By: Walter L. Dean

9781631871610

PUBLISHER'S NOTES

Disclaimer – Speedy Publishing, LLC

This publication is intended to provide helpful and informative material. It is not intended to diagnose, treat, cure, or prevent any health problem or condition, nor is intended to replace the advice of a physician. No action should be taken solely on the contents of this book. Always consult your physician or qualified healthcare professional on any matters regarding your health and before adopting any suggestions in this book or drawing inferences from it.

The author and publisher specifically disclaim all responsibility for any liability, loss or risk, personal or otherwise, which is incurred as a consequence, directly or indirectly, from the use or application of any contents of this book.

Any and all product names referenced within this book are the trademarks of their respective owners. None of these owners have sponsored, authorized, endorsed, or approved this book.

Always read all information provided by the manufacturers' product labels before using their products. The author and publisher are not responsible for claims made by manufacturers.

This book was originally printed before 2014. This is an adapted reprint by Speedy Publishing LLC with newly updated content designed to help readers with much more accurate and timely information and data.

Speedy Publishing, LLC©2014

40 E. Main St. #1156

Newark, Delaware

19711

Contact Us: 1-888-248-4521

Website: http://www.speedypublishing.com

REPRINTED Paperback Edition: ISBN: 9781631871610

Manufactured in the United States of America

DEDICATION

This book is dedicated to my wife Sarah. It was her who introduced me to the wonderful world of aromatherapy oils and I owe her my life for that. I never knew one could get so much healing and peace from the use of essential oils.

TABLE OF CONTENTS

Walter L. Dean

Aromatherapy- An Introduction

You have probably heard the term Aromatherapy and wondered what exactly that funny word, "aromatherapy" actually means. It is the use of plant oils in their most essential form to promote both mental and physical well being. The use of the word aroma implies the process of inhaling the scents of these oils into your lungs for therapeutic benefit.

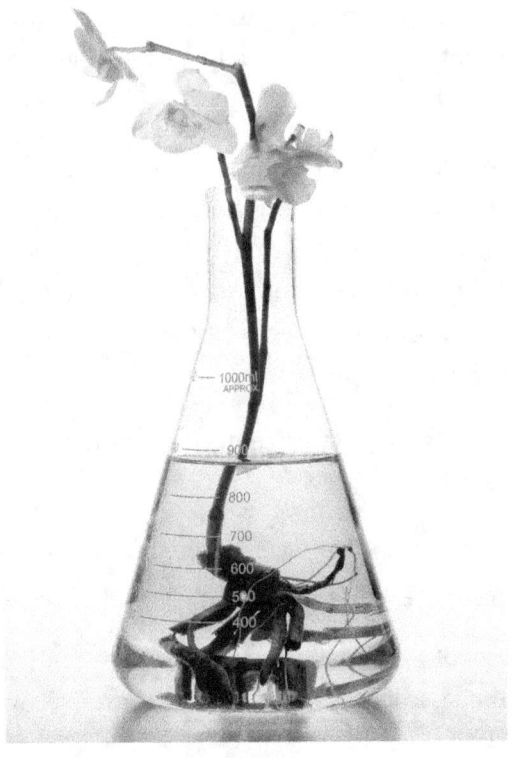

If you have ever used a vapor rub for a cough, then you have tried aromatherapy, although not in its purest form. As a matter of fact, you probably have been using aromatherapy on yourself and your family for many years without realizing it through vapor rubs or electric vaporizers.

Vicks or other brands of vapor rub use eucalyptus or menthol to clear up stuffy chests and noses. Imagine if you used the undiluted essential oil of eucalyptus how clear your lungs would feel.

The term aromatherapy is generally new, beginning to be used in the 20th century, but the practice has been around for thousands of years. It is believed that the Chinese were one of the first cultures to use the scents of plants to promote health through the burning of incense. Ancient Egyptians used distilled cedar wood oil mixed with clove, cinnamon, nutmeg, and myrrh to embalm the dead. The Egyptians also used oils to perfume both men and women.

In the 14th century, when the bubonic plague hit, killing thousands of people, the aromas were used to ward off the deadly disease. There is even discussion that the popular nursery rhyme, "Ring Around the Roses" refers to aromatherapy. The lines, "a pocket full of posies" allegedly refers to keeping the flower in one's pocket in an attempt to keep the illness away.

Moving forward through later centuries a growth in books about the use of oils in healing grew.

The Greek alchemist, Paracelcus, used the term "essence" and focused study on the use of plants for healing purposes.

While the use of essential oils for perfume continued to grow throughout the ages its" use for medicinal purposes waned slightly until around 1928.

It was at that time that a French chemist named Rene-Maurice Gattefosse accidentally discovered the use of lavender essential oil to heal wounds.

Walter L. Dean

The story is told that he burned his forearm and reflexively placed it in the closest liquid he saw, which was lavender essential oil. He was surprised to find that the burn healed rapidly and left no scar. It was then that he began using the term aromatherapy and wrote about the powers of essential oils.

Today, many people are trying to get back to nature. People have seen firsthand the dangerous effects of synthetic chemicals and processed medications.

The use of all natural essential oils for medicinal, cosmetic and therapeutic purposes continues to grow. Many people have found the results of using aromatherapy to be far greater than man-made medications and with far fewer negative side effects.

Aromatherapy can be used by itself or in conjunction with typical medical treatments. For example, you may use aromatherapy to ease pain after a surgical procedure. You still get the benefit of the surgery, but do not have to take the powerful and often dangerous pain medications that a doctor prescribes.

CHAPTER 1- HOW TO BE SAFE WHEN HANDLING ESSENTIAL OILS

Essential oils that are used in aromatherapy are not always easy to find. The Food and Drug Administration does not regulate essential oils so you, the consumer, will have to carefully read the ingredients of any oil you purchase to make sure that it is in its purest form.

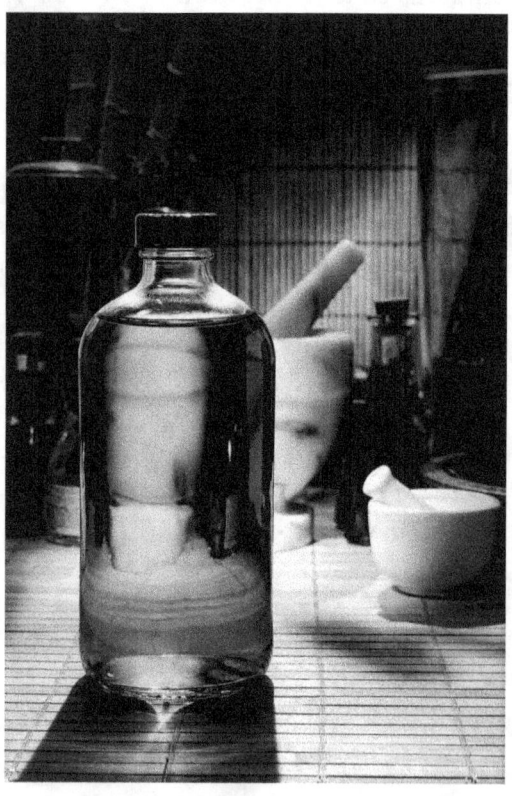

In order to get the most benefit from aromatherapy, oils in their purest form should be used.

Finding the Best Essential Oils

Try to avoid synthetic oils. Essential oils are the only way to get therapeutic benefit from aromatherapy. They will not be cheap nor should many different kinds of oils be priced the same as the process of distilling them is varied.

Light exposure decreases the ability of an essential oil to work, so only buy oils that are sold in dark bottles.

The term "oil" is often a misnomer as many of them are not at all oily. To test how distilled an oil is try dropping it on a piece of paper to see if it dissolves quickly and does not leave an oil spot.

If you have a health store in your area shop there instead of a perfume store. It is more likely that they will have real essential oils for sale.

Safety When Using Essential Oils

Essential oils are very powerful when they are not diluted. In order to make them safe you should dilute them with a carrier oil. Ask at your local health store which carrier oils they have available as there are many from which to choose.

Follow the instructions carefully when making any essential oil compound. If a recipe says one drop, use only one drop. Anyone who has a nut allergy should also avoid carrier oils derived from nuts.

Oils should be stored out of children's reach; if accidental ingestion occurs, contact poison control immediately. Pregnant women should consult their physician before partaking in any kind of aromatherapy.

If you plan to use aromatherapy for infants or the elderly it is recommended that you use lesser amounts of oil in your recipe. Check with your physician to ensure that it is safe to use on a particular age group.

Some oils can be toxic if ingested even in small amounts. In general, unless specified for oral use, essential oils should not be ingested.

Essential oils stored in a cool, dry place, and tightly capped will last six to twelve months. It is important to keep as little oxygen in contact with the oils as possible, so you will want to store them in full bottles, stepping down the bottle size as needed.

Essential oils should never be put on your skin in their undiluted form. They can irritate your skin quickly and cause a chain reaction that will make you sensitive to that oil for a lifetime.

Persons with asthma, epilepsy, or other serious health conditions should contact their physician before using aromatherapy.

To avoid an allergic reaction, place a small amount of diluted oil on a patch of your skin. Cover the spot with a band aid and wait a full day to see if irritation occurs. This can avoid a potentially large allergic reaction to essential oils. Essential oils should be kept away from open flame or fire hazards as they are all flammable. Never use any sort of oil near your eyes. Wash your hands thoroughly after handling essential oils to avoid contact with eyes or mouth.

CHAPTER 2- ARE ESSENTIAL OILS HAZARDOUS?

Some essential oils are very dangerous. These oils should not be sold at all, but can still be purchased over the internet or at less reputable shops.

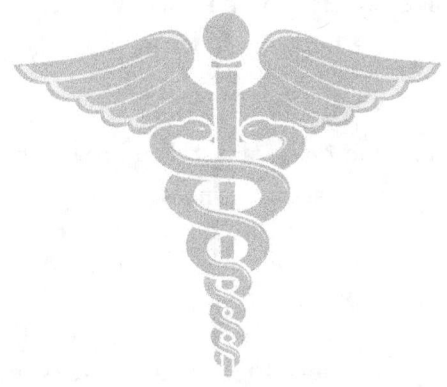

Others may be safe in some instances but can be rather dangerous if used in certain circumstances. Before you take on an aromatherapy plan, take time to understand which oils are safe. Keep in mind that just because something is all natural does not necessarily mean that it is not hazardous to your health.

- Rosemary, common sage, hyssop, and thyme should never be used if you have high blood pressure.

- Sweet fennel, hyssop, sage, and rosemary should be avoided if you have epilepsy.

- Diabetics should not use angelica.

- Those who suffer from hypoglycemia should stay away from geranium

- Sufferers of kidney problems should be cautious if they use juniper, sandalwood, or coriander.

- Expectant mothers should especially avoid juniper, hyssop, clary sage, peppermint, lemon, fennel, lemon verbana, rosemary, and wintergreen.

- Clary sage should not be used while drinking as it will intensify the effects of the alcohol causing it to act like a narcotic.

- Chamomile and marjoram should not be used while driving because they cause drowsiness.

- Some oils can cause allergies, such as citronella, clary sage, ylang ylang, and verbana oils.

- Oils that are believed to be carcinogens are calamus and sassafras, should be avoided by everyone.

- Methyl salicyalte is the active ingredient in aspirin and sweet birch essential oil. If you use aspirin for medicinal purposes you should avoid it due to the risk of overdose. It should also be kept away from children as it smells sweet and is equally dangerous to them.

While the list above outlines oils that can be dangerous in certain situations there are other oils that should not be used in aromatherapy at all. These oils can be caustic if inhaled and should be avoided at all costs. This is not a comprehensive list, you should do research on any oil you plan to use before you purchase it.

Oils That Should NOT Be Used In Aromatherapy

- Almond - Contains cyanide which even in small amounts can be lethal.

- Aniseed - Skin irritant.

- Arnica - Can cause dizziness and heart irregularities

- Bergamot - Phototoxic, severe sunburn could occur if it is exposed to sunlight.

- Boldo Leaf - Produces convulsions, even in small quantities.

- Calamus - Has carcinogenic (cancer causing) properties and can cause kidney and liver damage.

- Camphor - Oral ingestion can be toxic.

- Cassia - Skin and mucus membrane irritant.

- Cinnamon Bark - Skin irritant.

- Costus - Skin irritant.

- Elecampane - Classified as a serious skin irritant.

- Fennel - Can cause epileptic episodes.

- Horseradish - Eye, skin, nose, and mucus membrane irritant.

- Jaborandi Leaf - Oral toxin, skin irritant.

- Mustard - Skin and mucus membrane irritant.

- Spanish Origanum - Skin and mucus membrane irritant

- Dwarf Pine - Skin irritant.

- Brazilian Sassafras - Banned by the FDA as a carcinogen and can be toxic even in small amounts.

- Savin - Skin irritant.

- Southernwood - Toxic to the skin and if taken orally.

- Tansy - Can cause convulsions, vomiting, uterine bleeding, and death as a result of organ or respiratory failure.

- Cedarleaf Thuja

- Thuja Plicata - Can be a neurotoxin.

- Wintergreen - Can be a skin irritant, especially to those with an aspirin sensitivity. The oil itself is poisonous.

- Wormseed - Toxic to the liver and kidneys, suppresses heart function.

- Wormwood - Consumption can cause visual and auditory hallucinations and addiction. It can also cause convulsions and be a neurotoxin.

There are some essential oils that are highly toxic and should never be used in any circumstance.

Essential Oils to Avoid Completely

- Mugwart

- Pennyroyal

- Rue

- Sage

CHAPTER 3- AROMATHERAPY- A LOOK AT THE BASIC CARE KIT

If you are just beginning your journey with essential oils and aromatherapy there are a few oils that will help you get started. These are some of the easiest to find yet versatile essential oils. Not only are they used for therapeutic purposes, but can also be used in many other applications.

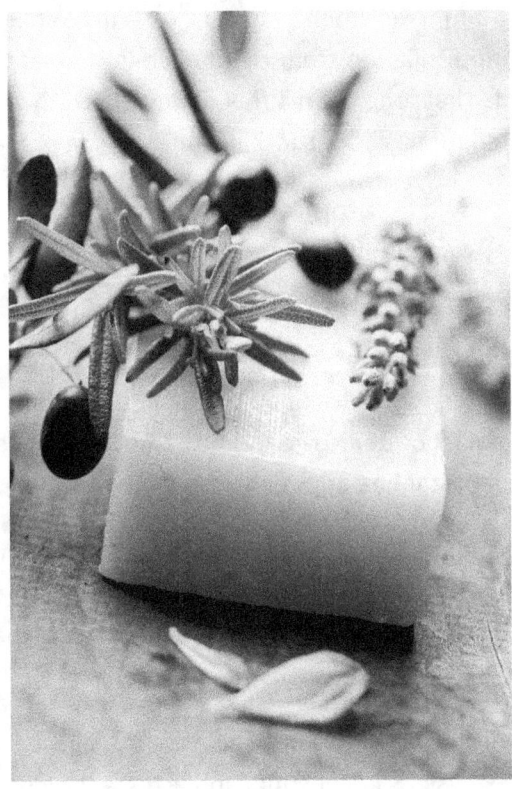

Some of these include making natural cleaning products and gardening. In addition to the oils you will need some way to get them into your lungs. An aroma diffuser is a good way to do this.

An aroma diffuser puts the essential oils into the air quickly and spreads them about the room which allows you to get your therapy by just relaxing and breathing deeply. They come in all different shapes and styles so you can purchase one that matches the décor in each room of your home.

Some run with the use of an open flame while others are powered by electricity. You can even get aromatherapy diffusers that work in your car.

Lavender

Lavender is a non toxic and non irritant essential oil. It is extracted through steam distillation from the flowering tops of the lavender plant. Lavender has long been a folk remedy used to calm an upset stomach. Lavender has both soothing and reviving properties.

Lavender oil should be clear to pale yellow and should smell sweet with floral and woody undertones. It blends well with other floral and citrus essential oils.

As aromatherapy it has a variety of health benefits. It's pleasant and calming scent makes it helpful in treating nerve and headaches, anxiety, depression, and emotional stress. It also increases mental stamina and calms exhaustion.

Lavender essential oil is often recommended to treat insomnia as its scent can induce sleep. Massage with lavender oil can remedy all types of soreness and pain even when it is deep in the joints.

The vapor form of lavender oil is used to treat all sorts of respiratory problems, including colds, flu, chest congestions, whooping cough, sinus congestion, and asthma. Lavender has been used to promote good blood circulation and stimulate the production of gastric fluids to treat stomach ailments.

Tea Tree

Tea Tree essential oil is also a non toxic and non irritant, but can cause sensitization in some people. This oil is extracted through steam distillation from the leaves and twigs of the Tea Tree.

Tea Tree has long been used by the aboriginal people in Australia and is named for their use of it as an herbal tea. The oil should be a pale-yellow, green or water white color. Tea Tree blends well with lavender, Clary sage, rosemary, and many spice oils.

Tea Tree oil is known for being anti bacterial, anti microbial, antiseptic, and antiviral. In short, it can almost be called a cure-all because it has so many properties to ward off disease and germs. In Australia it is found in nearly every household because of these properties.

Tea tree oil can be used as an antibacterial to cure all sorts of bacterial infections including the treatment of wounds. As aromatherapy it can be used to treat coughs, colds, congestion and bronchitis. It can also keep fungal infections at bay and even cure dermatitis and athlete's foot. Tea tree can be used as a stimulant to hormones and circulation and to boost one's immune system. Tea tree oil can help remove toxins by opening pores and promoting sweating, which removes uric acid and excess salt and water from your body.

Peppermint

Peppermint essential oil is nontoxic and when diluted, is a not irritant. It can cause some skin irritation because of the menthol properties it holds and should be used with temperance.

The use of Peppermint has been seen as far back as Egyptian tombs from 1000 BC. It also has a history of use in China and Japan since the earliest times to treat all sorts of health anomalies.

Peppermint essential oil should be pale yellow or greenish in color. It has a strong grassy mint scent. Peppermint works well with other mint scents like eucalyptus as well as rosemary and lavender.

Peppermint has been studied in the science community and its health benefits proven. Because of this peppermint oil is available in pill form. It contains many minerals and nutrients like iron, magnesium, calcium, omega-3 fatty acids, and Vitamins A and C.

Peppermint is an excellent remedy for respiratory problems and is widely used as an expectorant to remove nasal and respiratory congestion. As an aromatherapy it can be used to treat nausea, headaches, depression, and stress. It has also been known to treat irritable bowel syndrome. As a skin care product peppermint oil can improve oily skin and replenish dull skin.

Chamomile

Chamomile is a non toxic and non irritant. It is extracted through steam distillation of the flowering chamomile plant. Chamomile has been used for over 2000 years in Europe for medicinal purposes. The oil should be a pale blue that will turn yellow as it ages. It will have a warm, fruity, sweet smell. Chamomile blends well with lavender and geranium as well as sage and jasmine.

Chamomile is well known for its calming properties. So much so that it can be used in aromatherapy to treat nervous disorders, headaches, and migraines. It is also used to calm allergies and asthma. Many women use it for the treatment of PMS or to relieve a teething or colicky baby.

Eucalyptus

Eucalyptus is relatively new to the aromatherapy family as it has only been used for the past few centuries. It is a non irritant but can be extremely toxic if ingested.

It is colorless as an essential oil but has a distinct pine like scent. The essential oil is from the leaves of the evergreen eucalyptus tree that is native to Australia.

As an aromatherapy it is used to treat respiratory problems like sinusitis, nasal congestion, sore throat, runny nose, coughs, colds, and bronchitis. It is able to treat all of these ailments because it is antibacterial, anti fungal, and a natural decongestant.

Eucalyptus also has a cool and refreshing scent which makes it great for treating exhaustion and mental disorders.

Eucalyptus can also be used around the house as a room freshener, in making natural soaps, in saunas for its antiseptic properties, and even as in mouth wash or toothpaste.

Geranium

Geranium has many healing properties but can cause some sensitization and influence hormone secretions so it should not be used by expectant mothers. Geranium oil blends well with citronella, lavender, orange, lemon, and jasmine.

If used in aromatherapy Geranium oil is a great astringent. It promotes the tightening of muscles to keep skin from hanging loose.

It has anti bacterial and anti microbial properties to help stave off infections of many kinds.

The essential oil is also known to be a cytophylactic which means it encourages cell growth. It can also be used to treat many mental disorders like depression, anxiety, anger, and premenstrual syndrome.

Rosemary

Although Rosemary is considered non toxic and non irritant when diluted it should be avoided by epileptics, expectant mothers, and those who have high blood pressure.

The flowering tops of the Rosemary plant go through a steam distillation process to form the essential oil. It should be a clear or pale yellow liquid with a strong herb-mint scent. Rosemary is one of the first plants that was used for both food and medicine. In the middle ages, it was used to protect against the plague and to drive out evil spirits.

When used in aromatherapy Rosemary oil can help to boost mental stamina and increase brain activity. It can also treat depression, mental strain, and forgetfulness. When one inhales Rosemary they will immediately feel uplifted making it excellent for relief of fatigue. It can also clear your respiratory tract and relieve sore throats, colds, and coughs.

Around your home Rosemary can be used as an air freshener and bath oil.

Thyme

Thyme essential oil is extracted by steam distillation from fresh or partially dry leaves and flowering tops of the Thyme plant. The oil should be red, brown or orange in color. It has a spicy and pungent odor. Thyme was one of the first plants used in Western herbal treatments mainly for respiratory and digestive health problems.

Thyme is anti bacterial, when used in its aromatic form it can prevent bacterial growth in and outside of your body. It is able to cure lung, larynx, and pharynx infections without affecting the rest of your organs like prescription cough medicines. Thyme is also known to boost memory and to treat depression.

Thyme essential oil is used as an insecticide both around the home and on your body. It can also help in treating bad breath and body odor.

Lemon

Lemon essential oil is non toxic but, it may cause skin irritation so it should be used with restraint. Lemon oil is phototoxic so exposure to sunlight is strongly discouraged. In Spain Lemon is known as a cure-all being used for everything from fever to arthritis.

The oil will be a pale green-yellow color that turns brown as it ages. It has a light citrus smell and blends well with fennel, lavender, sandalwood, and chamomile.

Lemon is very popular for cooking and for its fresh scent. As aromatherapy it can aid in the relief of stress, anxiety and fatigue.

The scent of lemon helps to increase concentration and alertness and bring an overall positive sense to those who inhale it. Lemon has also been used in treating coughs and colds and it the treatment of asthma.

The high amount of vitamins in Lemon oil makes it an immune system booster. It can also improve circulation and stimulate white bloods cells further aiding one's ability to fight disease. Lemon has also been used as an aid in weight loss.

As a household cleaner lemon can be used on metal surfaces like knives to disinfect them; it can also be used in soaps and facial cleansers as it has antiseptic properties.

Clove

Clove oil should be used with extreme care. It can cause mucus membrane irritation and severe skin irritation. As such it should only be used sparingly and well diluted.

The buds, leaves, stems, and stalks of the clove plant are distilled with water to extract the essential oil. It should a pale yellow color with a spicy scent.

Clove mixes well with sage, allspice, lavender, and rose. Clove has been used all over the world for centuries. It can be used to season food as well as for medicinal benefit. Clove contains many minerals including calcium, iron, potassium, and vitamins A and C.

Clove has many health benefits, namely in the form of dental care. It has germicidal properties that aid in relieving tooth aches, gum sores, and ulcers in the mouth. It can also help relieve a sore throat.

Clove is an aphrodisiac which makes it a great stress reliever when used as aromatherapy. It can also have a stimulating effect and help to ease fatigue. Clove can also be used to treat headaches, bronchitis, asthma, coughs, and colds. Expectant mothers can use clove to relieve the nausea and vomiting often experienced during pregnancy.

Clove cigarettes have long been a popular alternative to the traditional tobacco kind. At one time it was thought that adding clove could counteract the negative effects of smoking, this has since proved false. The American Cancer Society notes that there is no scientific proof that clove cures cancer in any way.

Walter L. Dean

CHAPTER 4- HOW ELSE CAN AROMATHERAPY HEAL?

Approaching a medical condition by exploring the possibility of using aromatherapy as a solution is definitely worth the effort.

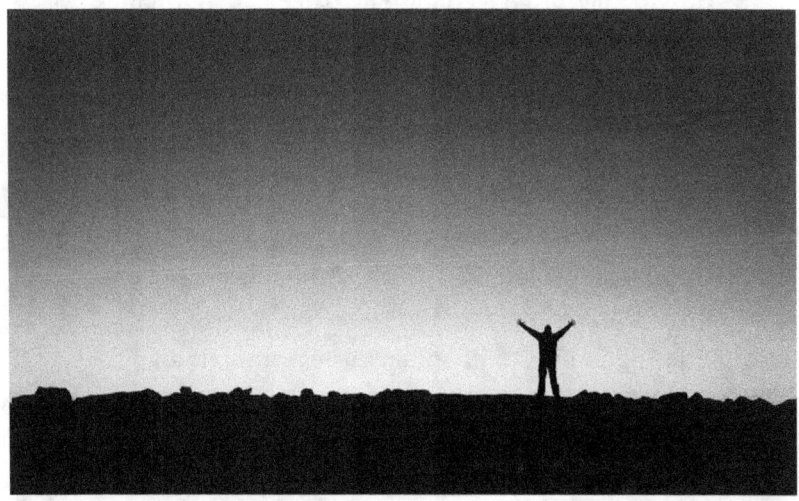

Aromatherapy ideally works when the psychological and physical aspects are addressed together. When the psychological and physical aspects are taken into account various contributing factors are studied carefully before any treatments are recommended.

The aroma therapist would have to consider factors like an individual's medical history, emotional condition, general health and lifestyle before putting forth any recommendations. This is a holistic style approach to treating a medical condition.

Applications

Some of the other more interesting conditions that are successfully explored using the aromatherapy method are backaches, irritable bowel syndrome, headaches and depression, to name a few. A good percentage of these medical ailments can be due to stress. Thus by using methods to understand and locate the individual's stress causing source, the aroma therapist will be able to alleviate the medical condition in a more efficient manner. In some extreme cases, claims of total recovery have been documented.

Treating skin problems is another avenue where aromatherapy has been successfully used. Conditions such as dermatitis, acne, eczema, psoriasis, cellulite, varicose veins and stretch marks are just some of the conditions where the use of essential oils has either arrested the condition or eradicated it completely.

Some patients have used aromatherapy to combat depression, hysteria, lack of concentration and panic attacks. Having tried other medically accepted methods which sometimes have undesirable side effects, aromatherapy has become a welcome solution. Treating burns, bruises and sprains using aromatherapy essential oils to achieve surprisingly quick and effective results are also another option worth exploring.

Other areas where the use of aromatherapy is being successfully explored are asthma, bronchitis, flu, and muscular aches and pains. When making the choice to use aromatherapy as a possible treatment for any given condition, it is important to ensure that only a qualified aromatherapy practitioner is consulted and that all the essential oils used are of the highest quality.

The popular belief that most illnesses and diseases are somehow linked to stress, anxiety and lack of proper daily nutrition has its merits.

Unfortunately some illnesses and diseases need to reach a critical stage before it becomes visible or is detected. To avoid all this, one is encouraged, though unrealistically, to keep all negative aspects in life under control or eliminate them altogether.

Wellness

Aromatherapy can helpfully contribute to this end. Primarily known for its calming properties, aromatherapy methods advocate the use of various essential oils to soothe the mind and body. Besides this a long list of other conditions can be successfully addressed with the use of aromatherapy elements.

Below are just a few examples of the capabilities and merits of using aromatherapy:

- Acne – lavender oil or tea tree oil to be applied directly onto the affected area. For milder cases, using a body bath lotion with these properties is recommended.

- Anemia – a concoction of tincture from the yellow dock root or an extract of dandelion leaf or even eating dandelion greens as a salad.

- Anxiety – chamomile, California poppy, passion flower, lemon balm

- Asthma – ginkgo biloba, mullein oil, a Chinese herb called shuan huang lian

- Bee sting – urtica urens , cantharis, lavender and vegetable oil mixed

- Body odor – alfalfa contains chlorophyll.

- Cold – eucalyptus oil in boiling water and inhaled. Gargle with a mixture of tea tree oil

- Cholesterol – chicory root, ginger

- Constipation – aloe vera juice, ginger tea

- Hair loss – saw palmetto, arnica, jojoba oil

- Headaches – chamomile relaxes, ginkgo biloba improves blood circulation

- Dandruff – flaxseed oil, primrose oil or salmon oil. Rinsing hair in chaparral or thyme

- Diabetes – huckleberry, tea made from most beans

- Diarrhea – blackberry tea, wild oregano

- Eczema – chickweed added to bath, stinging nettle, hazel ointment

- Indigestion – gentian root for better digestion, ginger, peppermint

- Nausea and vomiting – catnip leaves, chamomile flowers

- Menopause – for skin use geranium essential oil, orange blossom water, sandalwood essential oil

CHAPTER 5- WHAT ARE THE PROPERTIES OF ESSENTIAL OILS?

The properties of essential oils are what make them so beneficial. While most of them smell pleasant, that is just a by product of their real benefit. The term essential oil may sound simple, but they are actually complicated chemical compounds.

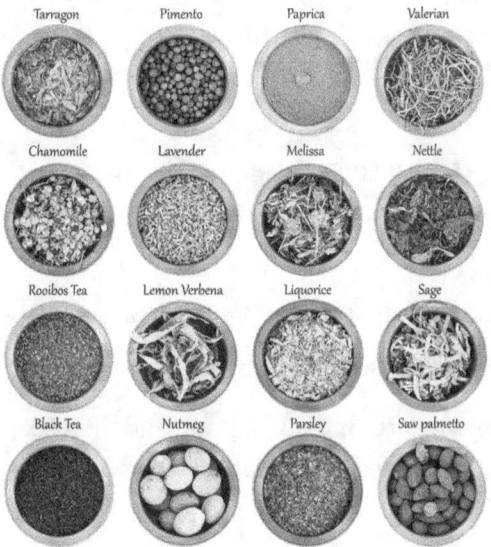

The ingredients in essential oils are organic because they consist of a molecule structure. This structure is made of carbon atoms and bound by hydrogen atoms.

In some essential oils there may also be oxygen, nitrogen, and sulphur atoms. By familiarizing yourself with the chemical makeup of essential oils you can understand how they might benefit your health. In turn you will also be able to understand why some oils are hazardous.

Main Chemicals in Essential Oils:

- Monoterpenes which have antiseptic and healing properties.

- Sesquiterpenes are anti inflammatory and anti infectious, they also have calming qualities.

- Phenols are a stimulant and best used in small quantities.

- Alcohols are antiseptic, antibacterial, antibiotic, and anti-fungal. They also stimulate ones immune system.

- Ethers are anti bacterial, anti spasmodic, and anti inflammatory.

- Ketones have relaxing and sedative properties. They are also an anti coagulant and can stimulate the immune system.

- Aldehydes can also be used as an anti inflammatory and to calm nerves.

- Coumarins are anti-convulsant and anti coagulative. They can also be used as a sedative.

Chapter 6- Aromatherapy Recipes for the Home

Remember that essential oils are very strong so follow each recipe with great care. Less is more when making essential oil treatments.

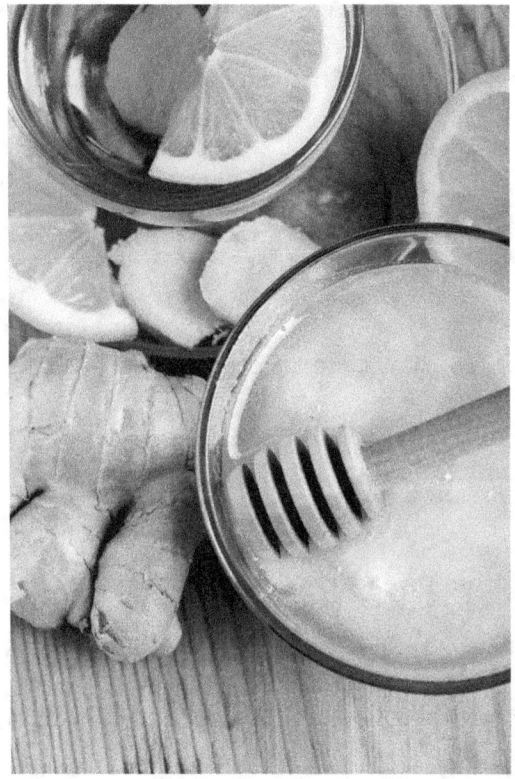

Diffuser Mixtures

For Attentiveness - 1 drop Cypress, 2 drops Cedarwood, 2 drops Lemon, 1 drop Pine.

For Recharging - 2 drops Fennel, 3 drops Juniper, 3 drops Lemongrass.

For Alertness - 2 drops Eucalyptus, 3 drops Rosemary, 3 drops Tangerine.

For Motivation - 2 drops Basil, 4 drops Bergamot, 1 drop Clove, 2 drops Ginger.

For Lucidity - 2 drops Bay, 3 drops Ginger, 2 drops Rosemary.

For Calmness - 2 drops Chamomile, 3 drops Lavender, 2 drops Marjoram.

For Harmony - 2 drops Benzoin, 2 drops Rose, 3 drops Verbena.

For Peacefulness - 4 drops Bergamot, 2 drops Clary Sage, 3 drops Cypress.

For Soothing - 2 drops Frankincense, 3 drops Melissa, 2 drops Patchouli.

To Increase Socialization - 3 drops Litsea Cubeba, 3 drops Rosemary.

To Relax - 3 drops Lavender, 1 drop Sandalwood.

For the Kitchen - 1 drop basil, 3 drops Lemon, 2 drops Rosemary.

For the Bathroom - 1 drop Basil, 3 drops Lemon, 2 drops Rosemary.

For the Bedroom - 2 drops Bergamot, 3 drops Jasmine, 2 drops Ylang Ylang.

For the Office - 2 drops Caraway, 3 drops Frankincense, 2 drops Ginger.

Home Cleaner Recipes

Walter L. Dean
Bathroom Air Freshener Spray

Fill a pump-spray bottle with 500ml of distilled water then add the following essential oils:

5 drops Cinnamon essential oil

5 drops Eucalyptus essential oil

5 drops Lemon essential oil

5 drops Sage essential oil

5 drops Thyme essential oil

10 drops Bergamot essential oil

10 drops Citronella essential oil

10 drops Lavender essential oil

10 drops Tea Tree essential oil

Shake this mixture well before each use. Spray every day to keep your bathroom smelling fresh and clean.

Lavender and Tea Tree Cleaner

1 teaspoon borax

2 tablespoon white vinegar

2 cups hot water

¼ teaspoon Lavender essential oil

3 drops Tea Tree essential oil

Mix all ingredients together and stir until dry ingredients dissolve. Pour into spray bottle for long-term storage and use. Spray as needed on any surface except glass. Scrub and rinse with a clean damp, cloth.

Disinfectant Spray

3 drops Cinnamon Leaf

5 drops Pine Needle

2 drops Frankincense

10 drops Bergamot

⅛ teaspoon Sunshine Concentrate

30 ounces water

Combine essential oils with Sunshine Concentrate and water in a 32 oz. trigger spray bottle. Spray on and wipe surface dry. It can be used to disinfect countertops, stovetops and tiles.

Microwave Cleaner

¼ cup baking soda

1 teaspoon vinegar

6 drops lemon essential oil

Instructions: Mix ingredients to make a paste. Apply to interior of microwave with a sponge. Rinse and leave door open to dry for 15 minutes.

Wash the glass turntable by hand. This recipe will get rid of food odors.

Floor Cleaner

¼ cup white vinegar to a bucket of water

10 drops lemon oil

4 drops oregano oil

Basic Wood Cleaning Formula

¼ cup white distilled vinegar

¼ cup water

½ teaspoon liquid castile soap

5 drops jojoba or olive oil

Combine the ingredients in a bowl. Saturate a sponge and squeeze out the excess. Wash surfaces of tired and dirty wood. The vinegar smell will dissipate soon. Dry with a soft cloth.

Creamy Soft Scrub

2 cups baking soda

½ cup liquid castile soap

4 teaspoons vegetable glycerin (acts as a preservative)

5 drops antibacterial essential oil such as lavender, tea tree, or rosemary

For exceptionally tough jobs spray with vinegar first—full strength or diluted, scented—let sit and follow with scrub.

Bath Recipes

Aromatherapy Bath Oil Recipe

2 ounces carrier oil like Jojoba

20 drops lilac Essential Oil or 15-20 drops of your own blend of essential oils (make sure they are EOs that are not known to be skin irritants)

Instructions: Blend the oils together and store in a glass bottle. The formula could be doubled or tripled.

To Use: don't utilize all 2 ounces of bath oil in one bath. After you've drawn your bathwater, add about ¼ ounce (7-8ml) of the bath oil blend to your water.

Mix well to ensure that the blend has scattered well in the tub and get on in. It's best to add the bath oil right before getting in the tub rather than while the water is running so that the essential oils don't vaporize before you get into the tub.

Utilizing this bath oil blend is safer than putting in pure EOs directly to the bath water. This is because pure essential oils added to bathwater may settle in one spot on your skin and cause aggravation.

Aromatherapy Bath Salts Recipe

3 Cups salt (Suggested salt types: Sea Salt, Dead Sea Salt, Himalayan Pink Salt, Epsom salt, or a combination of these salts). Salts commonly come in various grain sizes. Blending multiple grain sizes may make your salts more visually appealing. While chunkier salts frequently look prettier, bigger salts do take longer to break up in the tub and may be a little painful if you step or sit on some chunks that haven't totally broke up.

15-24 drops of your decided essential oil or essential oil blend. Make sure and take heed in the safety data for the oil(s) you decide to utilize.

Optional: 1 tablespoon Jojoba, Fractionated Coconut Oil or additional carrier oil for moisturization.

Instructions: Place the salt mixture into a bowl. If you've decided to include the optional oil inside your salt recipe, add it to the plain salts and blend well with a spoon or fork. And then, add the drops of your decided essential oils.

Once again, mix really well. Add the mixture to a pretty jar, salt tube, or container that has a tightly fitting lid. Salts that are kept in a container that's not air tight will lose their scent more quickly.

After a day, you might wish to mix well again to ensure that the oils are well blended.

To Color to Your Salts

For the rawest bath salt recipe, leave your bath salts undyed. Particular exotic salts including Hawaiian Red Sea Salt and Black Sea Pink Salt are by nature colorful. Try blending these salts with Dead Sea or plain sea salt for a flecked effect.

If you would like to add color to your salts, FD&C liquid dye or mica powder may be imparted before you add the essential oils. When putting in FD&C grade liquid dye, make sure to add only a drop at a time and mix well.

When adding mica powder, only add a flyspeck amount (1/16-1/8 a teaspoon is commonly sufficient) and mix really well. Utilizing too much dye or mica powder may discolor the water and discolor skin, so be really careful.

Leave bath salts at a soft pastel color. It's likewise crucial that you make certain that you're using skin-safe colorants and that the user of your bath salt blend doesn't have any allergic reaction or sensitizations to the colorant that you've selected.

To utilize: Add ½ 1 cup of the salts to running tub water. Blend well to ensure that the salt has scattered well in the tub prior to entering. To keep the essential oils from vaporizing too quickly, you may add the bath salts right before getting in the tub rather than while the water is running.

CHAPTER 7- USING AROMATHERAPY OILS TO SPICE UP ROMANCE

If used fully, our 5 senses heighten romance, love, intimacy and the meaningful times of our lives.

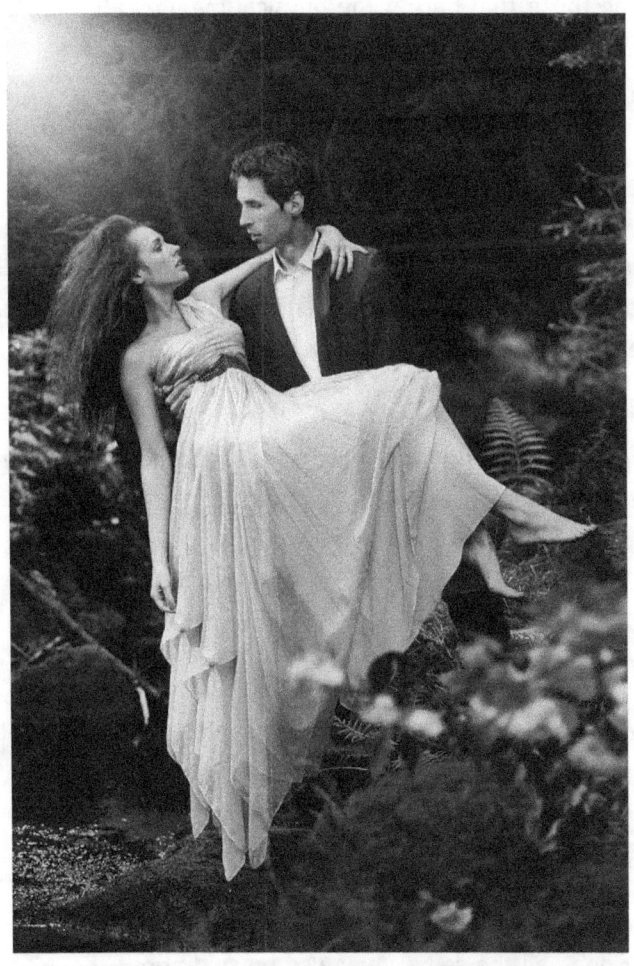

For Love

While the words sensuality and sensual are frequently misapplied, a sensual person is one that has an intense awareness and admiration of the subtle changes that impact each of the senses.

Such a person tends to value creativeness and tends to have an exceptional interest in activities that capitalize on the senses. Such activities include assorted forms of music, culinary innovations, the visual arts, aromatics and assorted forms of physical touch including those that permit the physical manifestation of love and desire.

Aromatherapy, natural botanicals and natural fragrance all tease our sense of smell. They play an important role within romance, love and intimacy.

Fragranced room sprays, body mists, bath oils, rub down oils, and additional natural aromatics may heighten a romantic evening or impart variety and intrigue to your union.

Including aromatherapy and natural aromatics in your plans for romance won't suddenly make a stubborn, unromantic and impassionate person get more loving or sensual, however, it may enhance his/her total mood, and make a romantic evening much more sensual. A room finely-fragranced with a fresh and exotic aroma may help melt away worries and lift up the spirit while setting the stage for the evening's plans.

Planning beforehand for special dates, evenings or additional times may help ensure a quiet (or interesting) beautiful occasion. Assigning special thought into all the aspects of a beautiful evening will make your mate feel special and prized, and will make the event unforgettable in his/her mind.

A great deal, all the same, may also be said about the advantages and wonders of spontaneous times. Impromptu moments may rule out including a few aromatic practices; however it's likewise possible to plan ahead for spontaneity. A lovely selection of natural aromatics may be bought or prepared beforehand so that you have them on hand for if the mood strikes.

An aphrodisiac is broadly defined as a substance that enhances or arouses passion and sexual arousal. Substances, including essential oils, that are thought of as aphrodisiacs are substances that may help disperse the physical, psychological or emotional ailments that might interfere with physical attraction or arousal.

CHAPTER 8- MISCONCEPTIONS ABOUT AROMATHERAPY

Confusing the attributes that come with using the term aromatherapy is mainly caused by the commercial sector seeking to capitalize in this area. For many people aromatherapy is usually linked to some pleasing scent emitted from essential oils.

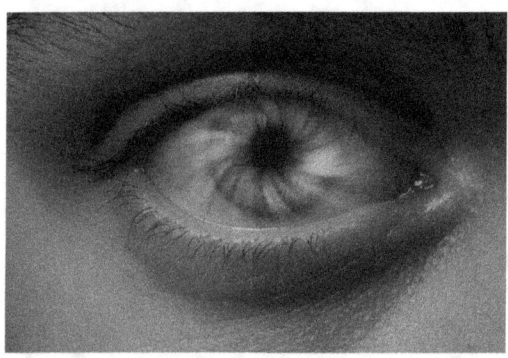

The effectiveness in the aromatherapy element is in the application and intent. Aromatherapy is meant to create a positive change physically, emotionally, mentally or spiritually, which is supposed to directly impact the body condition of the person undergoing a session.

However when products are touted to use or contain essential oils for aromatherapy purposes without actually comprising of the much needed dosage, it is no longer considered aromatherapy.

Aromatherapy or commonly referred to as the practice of using essential oils for medicinal and therapeutic purposes covers many areas of healing properties. There are many essential oils used as remedies for various physical conditions and complaints. Essential oils are also believed to contain anti-viral, anti-fungal and antibacterial properties. There are also some essential oils that work well for various skin problems.

Misusing Aromatherapy

The term aromatherapy has been so loosely used over the years for commercial reasons that it has become almost totally misleading.

Understood to mean a combination of two basic words – aroma and therapy, the word aromatherapy has been commercially used so widely that many false claims have been made over the years to promote and capitalize on it. A little time and research should shed light on this confusion.

Be Cautious

Aromatherapy is actually a serious foray to embark upon as it involves the use of pure essential oil and other natural ingredients that are considered safe to use only if done correctly. Not understanding the attributes and purity of aromatherapy, can lead serious repercussion as not all natural and pure oils are safe for human use. Some essential oils can even be toxic in certain circumstances.

Pregnant women and lactating mothers should be weary when choosing to use aromatherapy. The strong scents can be harmful to babies as their senses and immune system are not fully developed yet. Also some scents can be off putting to the baby and this may affect the baby's sleep patterns and feeding schedules, thus causing health issues from the neo natal stage.

Though aromatherapy has calming effects, using some essential oils to sooth and relax a cancer patient may have adverse effects. A doctor's permission should always be sought before trying this form of therapy. Some of the essential oils may have negative reactions to the prescription drugs already taken by the patient.

Made the choice to use aromatherapy as an alternative to other medical options, should only be done after extensive studies have been made of the advantages and disadvantages.

Although most illnesses and diseases are found to be the root cause of stress, anxiety and other pressurizing conditions, opting to treat the medical condition by using aromatherapy may produce minimal positive results to actually combating the disease or illness.

Overenthusiastic use or indulgence of aromatherapy can lead to serious problems, especially when medical advice has been ignored in making this choice. Some studies continually show little of no evidence in demonstrating efficacy against bacterial, fungal or viral infections, thus rendering it a poor alternative to medically proven alternatives.

In most countries around the world, the aromatherapy use is still related to the indulgent relaxing aspect. Hence there is no regulatory body that strictly governs the content and potency of each essential oil used for the aromatherapy session.

Undiluted essential oils used for aromatherapy can sometime cause skin irritations and discolorations. In cases where the natural product has been exposed to chemicals in their growing stage, such as pesticides, chemical allergies can have a negative effect upon application. In more severe cases the presence of estrogens like elements, have been found to negatively affect the delicate skin of children.

Some cultures take the aromatherapy influence to the extreme. Ingesting certain ingredients is widely practiced and sometimes causes severe irreparable damage. As some of the essential can be quite toxic when ingested, medical advice should always be sought before advocating such a choice.

As with any bioactive substances the method of aromatherapy, using essential oils, and while safe for the general public can still have adverse effects when used by pregnant or lactating women.

Some of the ingredients and methods used in a particular aromatherapy session may cause negative side effects when interaction with other more conventional medicinal elements are present. Adulterated oils used in some aromatherapy sessions can also pose problems depending on the type of substance used.

Other safety issues like the unsubstantiated claims made by those advocating aromatherapy as a proven alternative treatment can be misleading at best.

Watch Oil Quality

Poor quality oils severely lack the optimum benefits it promotes itself to have. In the course of processing these oils many factors should be considered if the end product is to provide what it promises to. Some of the things to consider are; if there are added chemicals, preservatives, substandard quality of ingredients, poor processing environments and adulteration of the oils. All these factors are important because harmful side effects can occur if other than the required essential oil is contained in the packaging. At best only minimal therapeutic benefits can be derived.

Some vendors combine the essential oils with other chemical and lesser grade ingredients for higher profit gains. These oils, then become either useless or less effective. Label words like fragrance oil, natural identical oil, and perfume oil are all words that are misleading in nature. As there are no strict guidelines to follow, some vendors intentionally or unintentionally use words like therapeutic grade or aromatherapy grade, thus these terms should be ignored and the contents examined closely.

Packaging styles are also another important factor to consider. Don't be misled by pretty packaging as it is the content that is important. Also essential oils that are packaged in darker colored bottles can be the way a vendor "hides" the clarity and purity of its content. The use of plastic style packaging is also not wise as some essential oils react with the plastic, thus causing the quality of the said oil to deteriorate considerably.

Chapter 9- Conclusion

The use of essential oils can be beneficial to your health. These products in their natural form promote overall well-being for those who use them.

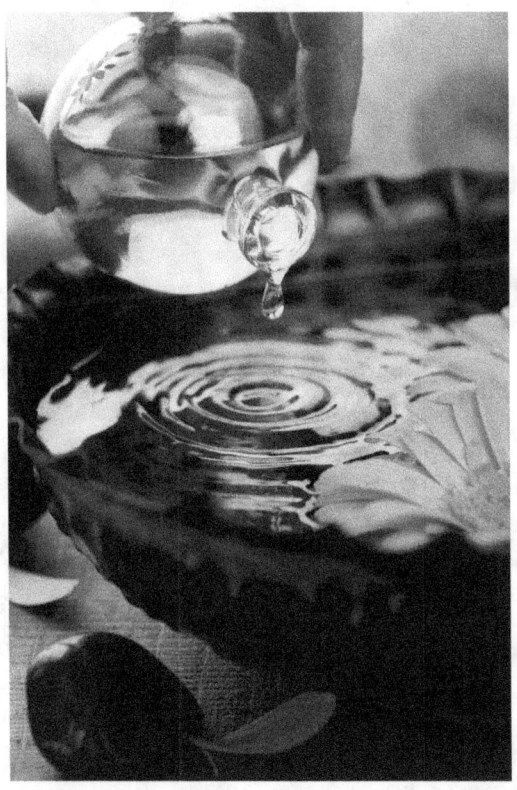

Instead of using complicated manmade chemicals, you use products what nature intended.

Not only can you maintain health but you can ward off illnesses like colds and flu just by inhaling lovely scents in your home, car, or office. The use of essential oils will improve your health and raise your energy level.

Aromatherapy: Healthy Complete Guide

Aromatherapy can even relieve tension and calm nerves. By using these complex organic compounds you can feel better and look better.

In addition to boosting your head to toe health the use of aromatherapy allows you to avoid using other dangerous products. When you use natures recipes to combat everything from diabetes to heart ailments you free yourself from the side effects of synthetic medications.

If you still require prescription treatment you can use aromatherapy in conjunction with them. Be sure to check with your physician before you mix any chemicals or if you are pregnant or have an ongoing health condition.

If you are just beginning your journey into the world of aromatherapy the kit listed here is a great way to get started. It provides you with commonly used oils that can be used in many recipes.

You should take time to familiarize yourself with the oils that can be hazardous especially as they pertain to your health issues or concerns. Remember that no two people are the same so what is a non irritant to another person may not be so for you. Simple tests can help you determine whether you will be allergic to oil.

As a novice to the field of aromatherapy you should also take note of safety precautions and hazardous oils. Some less scrupulous sellers, especially online, will still sell things that you should not use in aromatherapy. If you see something that looks suspect trust your research and avoid it.

Once you experience the benefits of essential oils you will wonder how you ever lived without them. Soon your home will be free of man-made chemicals for cleaning and treating illnesses.

Walter L. Dean

Do not underestimate the power of ridding your home of the scent of bleach and strong household cleaners. Imagine what taking those smells into your lungs does to your respiratory system. Now think of how it feels to breathe in fresh healthy air. This is what happens when you use essential oils to maintain a clean home. You and your whole family will be able to breathe easier and feel better. All of this by using natures essential oils through aromatherapy.

Aromatherapy is for you. It is meant to benefit your health and well being. All the tools you need are some high quality, natural oils and a few recipes. More important is the knowledge that you do not have to do harm to yourself to keep your body and home free of germs, bacteria, and negative energy.

So, find a health food store and start stocking up on oils that you like. Smell them all and see which invigorates you. Build a beginner kit and start healing yourself with essential oils. Once you do that your only job is to breathe.

ABOUT THE AUTHOR

Walter L. Dean went through most of his life being unaware of a lot of things. One of these things that he knew little about was aromatherapy. He had heard the term being bandied about but was not really interested in finding out any more about it. It was when he met Sarah, whom he later married that he started to learn the true benefits of essential oils.

He found that these oils could be used for just about anything from the common cold to helping with more serious problems. Walter became so proficient in the use of aromatherapy oils that he now helps his wife to spread the word on how useful they can be.

www.ingramcontent.com/pod-product-compliance
Lightning Source LLC
Chambersburg PA
CBHW071137280526
45787CB00003B/1313

* 9 7 8 1 6 3 1 8 7 1 6 1 0 *